Muchas Tortillas: FAT to PHAT

Muchas Tortillas: FAT to PHAT

Irma Concepcion Gonzalez Porter

ISBN: 154132918X
ISBN 13: 9781541329188
Library of Congress Control Number: 2016921447
CreateSpace Independent Publishing Platform
North Charleston, South Carolina

Acknowledgement

To the dedicated staff at the hospital, I would like to thank you for your professionalism and skillfulness with regard to my surgery. Special thanks go to Dr. Wisbach my surgeon, my dietician Eva and the excellent nurses. May God bless you and keep you in his favor.

Raised with my *familia*

You're about to hear the story of someone who overcame the struggle of being overweight a majority of her life. My hope is that it inspires you to find your true self. As a child I grew up in a traditional Mexican household. We were brought to the United States by our stepdad when I was seven years old and my brother was three. My mother was a tiny Mexican woman who knew how to cook great Mexican food, and when she cooked, she cooked everything—tacos, mole, refried beans, and flour tortillas. She cooked with lard and lots of salt; when she cooked sweets, she used lots of sugar. My mom made us *agua de arroz* or *horchata* (rice water) with lots of sugar. Because of the relationship my mother had with cooking, she instilled in me a serious relationship with unhealthy eating. I was not allowed to throw any food away, I was forced to eat everything on my plate, and oh, by the way, I enjoyed the unhealthy eating somewhat. Our family used food for bonding, and since our family was dysfunctional, we needed to do a lot of bonding. My mom was an alcoholic, so when she drank, she was a totally different person—not so nice. Those times I would turn to food; I ate to forget what was going on. Food made me feel good—I would hide somewhere and eat all kinds of food, mainly sugar. Food was my best friend; food never yelled at me or judged me. Food gave me a sense of well-being, even euphoria. In our household we didn't talk about our problems, and we were not allowed to tell anyone else. As a child, I was "the fat kid." Since I was never taught self-esteem at home, I was a loner and didn't like myself. (Even though Mom was actually a nice person when sober, she was a negative person when she was drunk—we were not close at all.)

When I went to school, I was always sad and depressed about my home life and about being the fat kid; I was always made fun of because of my weight. I remember two girls at school gave me the name *ballena sin cola* (whale without a tail). I hated that name, and it just made me go hide so I wouldn't have to be around them. I was always scared, and when I was frightened, I would do what I did best—stuff my face. That always worked. I remember that before I came to the United States, my brother and I used to go to the Catholic church because they always fed us. Once I ate so much that I threw up all the food, and even after I threw up, the nuns gave me a bag of food to take with me. Guess what—I ate it on the way home, then threw up again. Being in school here in the United States was so hard for me, because at first I didn't have any friends and didn't know how to make friends. Eventually, in grade school, I met a petite girl named Leela, and she and I became best friends. When we got to talking, we just didn't stop talking, and we found out she lived two doors from me. We loved playing with Barbie dolls and loved to play tag. We walked to school together and ate lunch together; she was so nice to me and accepted me for who I was. We often shared with each other our feelings of sadness. I remember once she said to me, "I wish I was a regular-size person; I don't like being a little person." My response was "You are a beautiful person inside and out, and I like you for who you are." I went on to add, "Really, don't worry about your size—you are fine, and you have a wonderful mom and dad who love you. I wish my mom was like yours—I would love for my mom to wake up in the morning like a regular mom, go to bed at a normal time, and not drink."

My favorite teacher was Mrs. Goodrum. She was so nice to me and would tell me I was a pretty girl and that I shouldn't forget that. She taught me how to multiply, and I remember when I first understood math. She was a great teacher. When I was in Mr. Dryer's class, he would have us go outside for physical education, and I would never participate because I was the fat kid. I was too embarrassed to do any activity because the other kids would make fun of me, so I always failed physical education.

When I was a child, my mother would take me to spend the weekend with my grandmother Concha. Before I immigrated to the United States, my grandma was the one that my cousin Chela and I spent the most time with. I loved my grandma; she was my father's mother. My grandma would tell me daily how much she loved me. She would put me to sleep by scratching my head. On Sundays she would take Chela and me to church, and I would always misbehave in church; all my grandma had to do was look at me, and then I would behave. My grandma taught me how to love. She would tell me daily that I was beautiful and I was a child of God. My grandma didn't have much money. My uncle Juan would sell flowers and also parrots at the international San Ysidro border crossing so he could support himself and my grandma. The little money he made would buy the food. My grandma would also make us eat everything on our plate, and we did. She would say, "*Comete todo hija no tenemos mucho dinero somos pobres.*" (Eat everything on your plate, honey—we don't have much money; we are poor.) I remember that when my grandma and Chela went to Juarez on vacation, I was so depressed—that's about the only time that I actually stopped eating. My mom didn't let me go on the trip with Grandma, and I was so sad. She and Chela were gone for about a month, and I lost weight, but as soon as she returned, I started eating and was the fat kid again.

My stepdad hated when I would spend time with my real dad, but I still saw my dad, Alex, anyway. When I was very young living in Tijuana, my mom and dad separated because my dad was in recovery from alcohol, and my mom was not ready for recovery, so they split up. I remember my dad would take me to his house with his new wife and my little brother and sister. We would go out to eat and watch television. I actually preferred my real dad over my mom anytime. I wanted to live with him because he loved me and was a good dad to me. I remember before they split up how mean my mom was to my dad, especially when she was drunk. She would always make him cry, and seeing that that would make me so sad. I remember the night he left—my mom and he had a big fight; he walked out and never came back home. I wanted my dad to be home with my little brother and me. I wanted him and my mom back together, but that didn't happen. I remember before coming to the United States when we lived in Tijuana, my mom would always leave my brother and me alone. One night my dad came by the house to see us; my father was angry that our mom was out getting drunk, so that night he took care of us, fed us, and loved us. The next day my mom finally got home drunk and was angry because our dad was with us, and she started another fight like always. My dad took us to my grandmother's house until she got sober enough to take us home. One night my mom had left again; she left a candle burning, and the curtains caught on fire. I remember there was a tiny window made out of wood right above the bed, and my baby brother was in his crib, crying. I remember he was wearing white pajamas, and I grabbed him by his feet and dragged him onto the bed. I then opened the tiny wooden window; the fire was getting bigger, with dark-orange flames. I crawled out of the window, grabbed my brother by his feet, and dragged him out. I left him on the sidewalk next to the window, ran upstairs, and got my aunt. She ran downstairs and, with another neighbor, put out the fire. My mom didn't get home till the next day. She really didn't react or seem to worry.

My mom met my stepdad when I was six years old. I didn't like him at first because I wanted my dad with us, but that changed. My stepdad took care of us and would buy our groceries. He was the one who brought us to the United States. I can remember so well the day we came across the US international border. I was seen by a doctor to make sure I didn't have any diseases. I didn't know any English, but I learned quickly. When I was six, I was skinny, but as I got older, I began to gain weight.

I remember when I was about ten years old, I went to Tijuana with my mom. I saw my uncles—Jesus, Juan, and Manuel—and my dad, Alex. They were crying, and my dad took me to the side, sat me down, and told me my grandma had died. I remember my cousin Chela and I couldn't stop crying, and we both had our arms around each other. I remember so well what she told me. As she cried, she said, "*No llores, hermanita. Manana te veo; te quiero mucho, hermanita."* (Don't cry, little sister. I will see you tomorrow; I love you so much, little sister.) We both were raised by our grandmother; she loved us both, and that day was one of the saddest days of my life. I remember returning back home to the United States and looking out the window every day, waiting for Chela to come see me. Days turned into months, and months turned into years. I lost all contact with my cousin. She and I were sisters; I missed her so much. I would never talk about my feelings. I would not say a word to anyone; I would just cry at night. I would eat and eat, and as I said in the beginning, food was my best friend and made me feel better. I remember when I graduated from the sixth grade, I was the chubby girl, and the day I graduated I wore one of my mom's dresses—I hated the way I looked. I started junior high school, and that was worse than elementary, because the kids didn't care if they hurt my feelings—they just called me fatty. I didn't have many friends in junior high. I was a loner like always, and I would run to food for comfort.

I finally graduated junior high and started high school. I was still the fat girl in school again. I didn't have many friends until I met my best friend Tammy; then it was her, me, and Mark, her boyfriend. We went everywhere together. She got me a job at a restaurant named Bonanza. Food was still my friend. I would always hide while at work, and eat the pie I was supposed to be selling. I still didn't have a good relationship with my mom. She never really knew where I was or what I did. With the money I made at Bonanza as a waitress, I bought my school clothes and bought my first car. Tammy and I would go to a club on the base named the Devil Dog Inn. We would go dancing every weekend at the marine base, and my mom never knew anything, as she was too busy drinking. Tammy was moving to Paradise, California, so we went out to the club that Saturday, October 19, 1985. Well, that is the day I met my husband.

I remember he sat next to me. I thought he was strange—he just sat there. I remember a song came on by Doug E. Fresh called "The Show," and I happened to love that song. He asked me to dance; I only danced with him because I liked the song. I gave him my phone number, and he called me a week later. I was so surprised that he called me—I was a fat girl, and I didn't think anyone would like me because I was fat. We began to date and went out every weekend. I was in the eleventh grade; I was seventeen, and he was eighteen. He was in the US Navy stationed on the USS *Constellation*. He then had to leave and go to Great Lakes for A school. After he left, he called me almost every day, and at that time there was no such thing as cell phones. We had one house phone, and I wouldn't let anyone touch the phone at a certain time of day because Markeith, my boyfriend, was going to call me. I remember that when the phone rang, I would run out of my room like a bat out of hell. We would talk on the phone for hours and hours. By this time I was working at Burger King to pay for school clothes and supplies. I remember trying out for the drill team and not making it. I was so embarrassed, but I was the flag girl and still wore the drill-team uniform. My teacher was Mr. Mitchell, a great teacher who loved his job and his students. I started making friends when I entered high school, which was great for me. I was still the fat girl in school, but I was accepted by my friends. I graduated in June 1986, and I remember my mom and stepdad not wanting to go to the graduation. I was devastated, but my friend Mickey from Burger King did go—he was also one of my best friends and one of the nicest people I have ever met. The only reason my mom and dad went to my high-school graduation was because my brother convinced them to go. In January 1987, Markeith returned to San Diego from the Great Lakes. My life was in transition—I was becoming an adult.

Youth to adulthood

In this great transition, my life was more of the same. My boyfriend, Markeith, told me how much he loved me and that he didn't care whether I was fat or not, because he loved me for who I was. I remember going to the airport because he was on his way home. I was so excited to see him—I hadn't seen him in two years. When we saw each other, we just kissed and hugged. I knew I was going to be with him forever; he was my soul mate. I remember going to see him at the barracks and we would go on dates every weekend. One weekend his roommate said he was going to be gone the entire weekend, but he came back that same night and caught us in bed together; we were both so embarrassed. A month passed, and I missed my period. I went to the clinic, had a pregnancy test, and found out I was pregnant. That night I saw Markeith and told him I was pregnant. I said to him, "I'm pregnant. My mom is going to kill me. We have to get married."

He said, "OK." We eloped and got married on January 24, 1987, and then searched for a furnished apartment in Chula Vista.

Three months later I told my mom and dad, "I'm pregnant, married, and moving out." I told them both all in one swoop. My parents were so pissed off. I remember I was so happy when I moved out—I was away from my mom, and I was relieved. I was getting bigger by the month and was induced on October 3, 1987. We had a little boy and named him Markeith J. Porter.

My husband left a month later to a six-month west pack and returned when my son was six months old. After I had my son, I really didn't lose that much weight, so when my husband left, I went to a weight-loss clinic, got myself some diet pills, and lost all kinds of weight. When my husband got home, I was skinny—not because I lost weight the healthy way, but because I was taking diet pills. Of course, I soon gained all my weight back...and then some! We would eat out all the time, and we loved our unhealthy way of eating. I was now a fat adult and never exercised; I just wanted to eat and feel good. My husband, my son, and I just did a lot of family things, especially going to my mom's house to eat. We then moved to Long Beach for a year because my husband got stationed there, and I worked as a cashier at the Navy Exchange. We moved back to San Diego and found out my stepfather had COPD; my stepfather then got very sick, and died of complications of emphysema. We were all very sad, especially my mom—she had lost her best friend. She then moved into the apartments my aunt owned. My husband and I then bought our condo, and my mom and brother moved in with us for the next year. While my mom lived with us, she cooked every day. Man, did she cook great food. She had the house clean every day. Since had I left home, I had missed coming home from work to my mom's cooking. I went to school to be an LVN (licensed vocational nurse), and graduated in 1991. I loved my job as a nurse and worked in many places. I was in a car accident in 1992 and was in the hospital for a month. Then, a month after I got out of the hospital, I got pregnant; nine months later we had a baby girl (May 17, 1993), and we named her Sabrina Armida Neshae Porter. I was so happy we finally had a little girl.

Again, I didn't lose that much weight after the birth; I was fat and hated myself. I went on fad diets to lose weight but soon gained it all back. I stayed fat for the next seven years until, in 2002, I decided to lose weight again. The diet program allowed one to count points. This facilitated how much intake of food was consumed in one day. I counted points; I loved this program, and it taught me a lot. At this point I weighed 135 pounds, and I kept the weight off for about seven years.

Unfortunately, then I stopped exercising and started overeating again—I gained all my weight back, and then some because I was stressed out at work and depressed. At this point, I just didn't care anymore. I didn't take many pictures, because I didn't like how I looked. I would exercise from time to time, but I was in denial about starting to gain so much weight again. I wish today that I had taught my children about healthy eating, but I didn't. I got so heavy that I was having a hard time breathing; I couldn't walk too far because I tired so easily. In fact, even the people I was employed to take care of seemed to be concerned about my shortness of breath, saying, "Why are you having such a hard time breathing?"

My answer was always, "I'm fine. Nothing is wrong with me."

Actually, I knew deep down inside they were so right, but I just didn't want to admit it. I can recall when there was a time when I took my kids shopping with me, and I had the nerve to try on a pair of pants that were way too small and tight. I asked my daughter how they looked; she just looked at me in shock, and when she told me that the pants were way too tight and that I needed a bigger size, I was so angry. She told me the truth, and I had the nerve to yell at my baby; then she was too scared to say anything to me after this incident. My family and I would go out to eat almost every night, and I would always eat extra food when no one was watching.

Hispanic population obesity rate

Obesity in the Hispanic population is on the rise. There are several diseases associated with the rising obesity rates. Among these are heart disease, diabetes, hypertension, strokes, and cancer. These diseases are associated with grave fiscal cost. In 2009 64.4 percent of the Hispanic population was considered overweight or obese (CDC website). In 2009 I lost my father, who had a massive heart attack. Though my father was not a large man, he suffered from heart disease and diabetes. I was so saddened by his death; I thought he would live forever, because he was such a strong man. My father actually drove himself to the hospital and died in the emergency room. My fondest memory of my father was when I was seven years old, and he took me to the beach. He bought me ice cream, and we just walked around feeling the breeze of the blue ocean and looking at the beautiful waves (this is the time when my father was in recovery). I loved my father so much. He was everything to me, and I will never forget him. I know he is watching me from up above.

My mom was a tiny one-hundred-pound Hispanic woman with a huge amount of spunk. She also suffered from heart disease, diabetes, and colon cancer. In October 1997, my mom was feeling sick and had been having diarrhea, so we called 911 and she was taken to Mercy Hospital. This is when we received devastating news: the doctor told my family and me that she had colon cancer and had only eight months to live. We were all in shock, sad, and in denial. My mom and I were never close, but this news actually made us closer. I can't believe what it took for us to get close. I now wish things could have been different. If I could go back in time, I would change so many things, but I can't.

After my mom got out of the hospital, she was living her life just like any other day. My kids, my mom, and I would drive over to the beach and watch the ocean. My mom loved the ocean, and she loved when we drove around just for the hell of it. I really think we all were in denial because no one ever spoke of her having colon cancer. Two weeks before she died, my mom and I got into a big argument. I stopped talking to my mom; looking back now, I realize that's the biggest mistake I've ever made. One afternoon my mom called me and asked me if I could pick her up at the bar. I told her I was on my way. My mom looked so sad; she had this look on her face, and this just tore me up inside. After I dropped her off at her apartment, we hugged, and she cried.

The very next day, my mom ended up in the hospital again with a massive stroke; the doctor told us that her cancer had also spread. The day after that, my mom went into a coma, and since she didn't have an advance directive, she was placed on life support. The doctor asked our family what we wanted to do. I told him that she didn't want to be on life support, and she was taken off. I was with my mom that whole day, and I saw her being taken off life support—she had tears falling down her face, and I also couldn't stop crying. I sat there and told my mom how much I loved her and how sorry I was for not being with her the last two weeks of her life. I saw my mom take her last breath. Our family was there with her, and we were all in tears. My mom had a beautiful funeral and it was a celebration of her life. I know my mom and I had a rocky relationship, but no matter what, I loved my mom—I wouldn't have traded that for anything in the world.

My husband also suffers from hypertension and takes medication. For myself I do not want to have to take medication for the rest of my life. By eating the right kinds of food and getting proper exercise, I hope to reduce my risk of getting one of the diseases associated with obesity.

The decision to have bariatric surgery

In December 2015, while shopping at the grocery store, I happened to bump into an old colleague of mine. When I asked her how she was doing, she told me she was having medical problems with her diabetes. Due to complication with diabetes, the doctor recommended gastric bypass surgery. The next day, I made an appointment with my doctor to discuss my options of having bariatric surgery.

When I finally saw my doctor, he gave me a referral so I could learn more about the types of surgeries available and to see if I qualified. I then received a call from the Naval Hospital about the referral my doctor had sent in for bariatric surgery. I was sent a questionnaire to bring with me to my appointment at the nutrition clinic. I attended a bariatric information session in December 2015. There were so many people there, and we were all there to learn about the different types of weight-loss surgeries available to us.

The first one that was presented by one of the surgeons was the gastric bypass. In the gastric bypass (GBP), the stomach and small intestine are rearranged in one of several different ways, the abdomen is separated into a small upper pouch and a much larger lower "remnant" pouch, and then any GBP leads to a marked reduction in the functional volume of the stomach, accompanied by an altered physiological and physical response to food (Hacker, 2011). The next surgical procedure presented was the gastric sleeve. Gastrectomy is a surgical weight-loss procedure in which the surgical removal of a large portion of the stomach along the greater curvature produce a reduced stomach functional reaction to about 15 percent of its original size., of the stomach, although there can be some dilation of the stomach later in life. The sleeve procedure is generally performed laparoscopically and is irreversible (Hacker, 2011). I decided that I wanted to have the gastric sleeve because I didn't want my intestines reconnected, and the sleeve seemed to me to be less intrusive than the gastric bypass.

Presurgery

I had so much to do to prepare for surgery, and I felt like I had such a short time to do it in. In phase one I had to complete the Nutritional Needs Education Class 1. This class provided information about the diet plan after surgery. The next class was the Bariatric Pre- and Post-Op Education Class 2. In this class we discussed perioperative expectations and general surgery. I also had to attend one pre-op support group meeting and a nutrition consultation. Next, I had to attend a series of three healthy-lifestyle classes. I also had to lose 10 percent of my weight, which was twenty-three pounds. I had to start a written food journal and physical activity log. I needed to see a psychiatrist for a consultation. I had to do a sleep study, a pap smear, a mammogram, and a colonoscopy. This concluded phase one.

Phase two

Phase two went a lot more quickly than phase one. I had to complete an upper GI study, a gallbladder ultrasound, a chest x-ray, blood and urine tests, an upper endoscopy, internal medicine and cardiology consults, and finally a pulmonary consult. Each hospital where weight-loss surgery is done has its own rules and policies on what has to be done prior to weight-loss surgery. I was placed on a strict fourteen-day pre-op diet of protein shakes, a very low calorie intake, and an exercise plan, so that I could lose as much weight as I could before surgery. Two days before surgery, I was on a full-liquid diet, which was difficult. Finally, after completing everything I listed, I was able to see the surgeon, and my surgery was set for May 18, 2016.

Surgery and postsurgery

On my surgery day, I was scheduled to have the gastric sleeve procedure at noon. The day before, I was so nervous but also excited about my new journey. The surgery took longer than expected (six hours instead of the three to four scheduled). The doctor said he had had a tough time with lesions, which had caused a bruise to my liver. We made it out of surgery, and it appeared to be a success. I was taken to recovery for two hours, then to my room. The next day I was brought a tray with all liquids, and I had a hard time drinking everything—it just seemed like so much to drink. I also had to start walking right away, even though I had so much pain and fatigue. Right after my surgery, I felt like maybe this was a mistake, because of the way I was feeling physically. I also found out during my sleep study that I have severe sleep apnea. During the sleep study, I actually stopped breathing eighty-seven times in one night, so now I use a CPAP machine during the night to breath. I had an incentive spirometer, and it was the hardest thing I had to do, because it was just so hard to breathe, but little by little I got better at it, and stronger. I was in the hospital for about three days and then was released to go home.

For the next two weeks, all I could take was fluids, which included protein shakes, broth, Jell-O, and more Jell-O. I got so sick of having the same thing all the time, and I was having such a hard time because I had to drink everything so slowly. I was also having diarrhea and I hated this. During this phase I was always so tired and had no energy. I was regretting having surgery, and I kept telling myself that I had made a mistake. I then saw my dietician and the doctor for my two-week checkup and was placed on soft pureed foods. I was so happy to go home and try something different. By my sixth week after surgery, I was taking about 120 grams of protein and was also taking vitamins; I had such a hard time swallowing my vitamins, but I did. By my third and fourth week, I was on pureed soft foods; by the fifth and sixth week, I was eating a little more solid food. By week seven I was eating a modified regular diet, and I was already losing so much weight.

When I began my weight loss journey, I weighed 230 pounds. The day of surgery, I weighed in at 191 pounds. I was so happy to have surgery. I know when I mention my weight I make it sound like it was easy to lose, but actually I was having such a hard time. After surgery I couldn't drink with a straw; I had to eat very slowly, and it seemed to take me forever to finish everything. I made sure to drink at least thirty minutes after I ate, and I would never drink while eating. I was very lucky that I never had nausea or vomiting, because I did what the dietician and my doctor told me. I didn't exercise until after I saw my surgeon for my sixth-week checkup. When I asked him when I could expect to get all my energy back, he told me it would come back, but that I had to be patient. I started to get my energy back during my third week, but still felt tired. I finally had my energy back at around my seventh week.

I also know that everyone is different—I learned never to compare my weight loss to some else who was losing weight faster than I was. I made sure to take all the vitamins that I was required to take by my doctor's orders. I also made sure to take my protein, because I knew at some point my hair would start falling out, and that is one thing I feared. So I drank my protein, always buying protein that I enjoyed (and still enjoy today). I also made sure to eat and drink sugar-free products. When buying protein, I made sure to follow the guidelines my dietician and doctor gave me. I made sure to exercise every day (walking and elliptical trainer), starting with thirty minutes a day, and increasing little by little.

My support system

When I started to consider having weight-loss surgery, the first thing I wanted to do was consult with my husband. I was scared, because I didn't know how he would react. When I told him, he said he loved me just the way I was, but if I wanted to have weight-loss surgery, he would stand by me. When I found out that I had to lose 10 percent of my body weight in order to qualify for surgery, I was stressed out. I told my husband that I didn't know if I could actually do it alone, and that I worried whether I was even going to lose one pound. To lose the weight, I started a program of walking and healthy eating, and my husband joined right in. We were doing weekly meal planning, and I just loved it because I was not doing it alone. I had someone losing weight with me—my husband whom I just love so much. He was, and still is, my main supporter. We both supported each other. I lost not just 10 percent of body weight, but a lot more

I then began searching for support groups on the Internet. I found a support group that is now one of my favorites. What I like about the site I found is that there are so many people just like me, with whom I could share my thoughts and my progress. I also love the protein shakes, food, and snacks. I know there are many people out there who feel alone because their families do not support weight-loss surgery. Please don't. I know it's not easy. For those out there who are feeling like this and do not have the support of their loved ones, there are many support groups in the community, at the hospitals that provide bariatric surgery, and on the Internet. You will be surprised at how many people are going through what you're going through. Go out there and meet other people with weight problems. Tell them about yourself; make friends and get phone numbers. Find walking buddies or even gym buddies. Do not be afraid. Before you know it, you'll see how much better you feel about yourself, and your new friends will feel the same way. Who knows—maybe your loved ones will even come around. I go to support groups at the end of every month on Tuesdays. When I first started going to the support groups, I met many men and women who inspired me with their stories about their weight loss. I had so many questions, and they were answered. I also heard so many stories. I remember a woman talking about when her hubby had come home from being away for six months—he had walked right past her and hadn't recognized her. When he did, he had been shocked, but happy and proud of her accomplishments. After hearing those stories, I told myself that I, too, was going to lose the weight; I felt inspired by attending these support groups.

For those of you out there who don't have the support of your families, there are other support systems available besides the ones I've already mentioned. For instance, I also use the church as a support system. This may not be your preference, but the church community has helped me; the women I have met have been so supportive. One church member in particular has been nothing but a positive reinforcement to boost my self-esteem. Those of you who have a church that you attend may want to look into meeting new friends and even finding men's or women's groups there. Even those of you who do not normally go to church can still use the church as a support system if you wish. In addition to church, there may be support systems available in the workplace. In my current workplace, one of my colleagues also lost weight—not through surgery, but through a diet program at a hospital; she looks amazing. We frequently talk about the progress we have both made, and this is another way to find support. You may also want to try creating your own support group at home or even at a local park. You will be surprised at how many people would attend your group. In your own support group, you have the ability to set the policies and tone of your meetings.

Me today

The decision was made, the surgery was done, and my initial weight loss is over. Starting out at 230 pounds, today I have finally reached my weight goal of 131 pounds. I have to take a total of twelve hundred calories a day to maintain. I keep my carbs at no more than fifty grams per day; when I was losing weight, I kept them between twenty-five and thirty-five grams per day. In the morning I usually eat egg whites with tomatoes and cheese; for my snack I will have a protein shake with one cup of sugar-free cashew milk. Then for lunch I have a pack of tuna salad with cheese and a slice of whole-grain bread; for my afternoon snack, I have turkey roll ups with a slice of cheese. For dinner I usually eat three to four ounces of salmon, tilapia, or lean meat and half a cup to one cup of vegetables. And for my after-dinner snack, I will eat a tiny piece of banana with powdered peanut butter. I log everything I eat and drink; I use an app that shows me how much protein, carbs, calories, and sugar to take in daily. I make sure to eat a total of twelve hundred calories a day.

I also do my daily exercise. I always take my hubby with me or take a friend along—that way my time goes by fast. One thing I love doing is hiking. We have found many hiking trails that are a lot of fun, and I take my phone so I can hear my music. I also have a pedometer that tracks how much I walk, which is so helpful. I am not the person I was before I had the gastric sleeve. In the past I would sit at home with my hubby, and we would eat and watch television. My hubby and I never did any type of physical activity, and I was always out of breath. My favorite foods to eat were any high-calorie foods. We loved to just sit around. I would be too afraid to weigh in until I finally got the guts, and I was so shocked.

I love who I am today, and I love my sleeve. What I love doing is shopping for clothing and trying on different outfits, especially outfits that I would never have worn in the past. I remember trying on a leopard-skin dress—I couldn't believe how good I looked, and I couldn't believe that was me in the mirror. I loved the person who was looking back at me in the mirror. I can actually say I have so much confidence today.

Last week my hubby and I went to church. We were in the parking lot, and a man was staring at me. I didn't know he was starring until his wife slapped him. I felt bad for him, but I did feel good inside—that is the truth. Once, after a misunderstanding in the parking lot of a grocery store, an angry woman called me a skinny-assed bitch, which I took as a nice compliment. When I ran home to tell my hubby, he told me I was crazy and laughed. My husband has noticed my confidence change; he feels all the extra happiness I have from my weight loss. Not only did I lose weight, but my hubby also lost a total of fifty-six pounds. I didn't do this all by myself—I had the support of my hubby—and this also benefited him because he is also eating and staying healthy with me. I still attend my support groups when I have the chance, because I have met so many inspiring women there. I love my online support group also. I do buy my protein shakes online, and they are delicious because there are so many flavors. I love the protein bars and microwavable pork rinds that are low in calories and high in protein. I make sure to take my recommended amounts of vitamins, minerals, and protein.

When I was losing weight I had some hair loss. but I was reassured by my dietician that it would all grow back, and it has. I recently went back to work. I am a nurse, and I love what I do. I make sure to take my break and eat outside. I make sure to chew slowly, and I don't drink until at least twenty to thirty minutes after I eat. I never drink any carbonated drink. This is one of the things I learned early on: my stomach is so small I wouldn't be able to tolerate carbonated drinks, and this does not bother me at all. I put water enhancers in my water (I buy different flavors).

Reflection

My weight loss has been truly fabulous and it has been great to focus all my energy on a plan to lose weight. I developed a mission and a vision that led to a considerable amount of weight loss.

The decision to have weight-loss surgery was not taken lightly. The risks of surgery had to be taken into account. I made my decision after talking with the doctors, nurses, and dietician. I was impressed with the thoroughness of the hospital program.

In the beginning of the book, I mentioned that I was thoroughly checked before the gastric sleeve procedure, and I was made knowledgeable about the different weight-loss surgeries and programs. My vision was that I would be healthy and fit. The journey from 230 pounds to 131 pounds has made me more self-confident. My mission was to develop a plan that included diet, exercise, and support. My diet plan includes protein, protein shakes, complex carbohydrates, and sugar-free foods, among other healthy foods. Daily exercise for thirty minutes to an hour has been important. Finding support has been a great part of my plan. My husband's support has been superb, and my support group has been the same. One of the things people don't take into account today is the impact of technology. My support group is online, and we post before-and-after pictures to help others know that they can achieve the same result. It is not easy, but anything that is worth having is worth working for. The other thing I do online is keep track of my calorie intake and exercise. It is most rewarding when you get to see a graph of your weight loss. This is very reaffirming.

So in my reflections, what I want you to take away from this book about weight-loss surgery is that, as with any endeavor, you must develop a plan that includes a mission and vision. The plan must be communicated to all stakeholders, and a decision to have or not have the weight-loss surgery must be made. If you decide to have the weight-loss surgery, you must be focused. You must focus on your diet, exercise, and support. Lastly, you might want to make technology an important part of your weight-loss plan.

So what is the title about? *Muchas Tortillas* is about a young Hispanic woman who, despite all the adversity she encountered as a child, was able to fight and win the battle of the bulge. Some of you may think, "How awful—she took the easy way out." I say you are wrong. I say there is nothing easy about following an eight-hundred-calorie-a-day diet. I say there is nothing easy about exercising one hour a day. There is nothing easy about understanding your support system and living with the one you have been provided. There is nothing easy about having surgery and the pain of recovery. So on a happy note, I was able to go from fat to phat. From me to you, go and make your *muchas tortillas* a reality for yourself and your family.

References

Hacker(2011). In Merriam-Webster.com.Retrieved Jan 6, 2017, from https://www.merriam-webster.com/dictionary/hacker